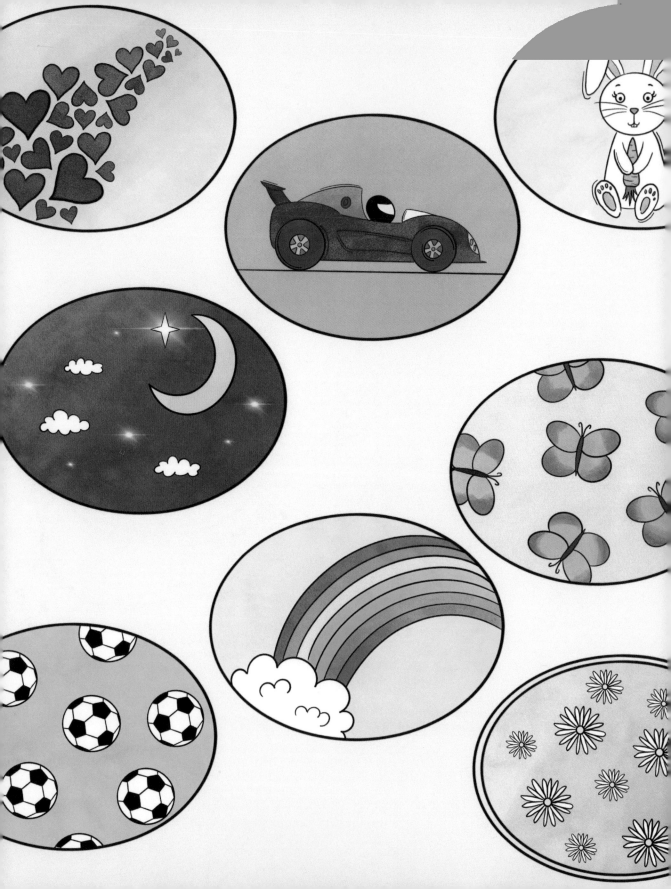

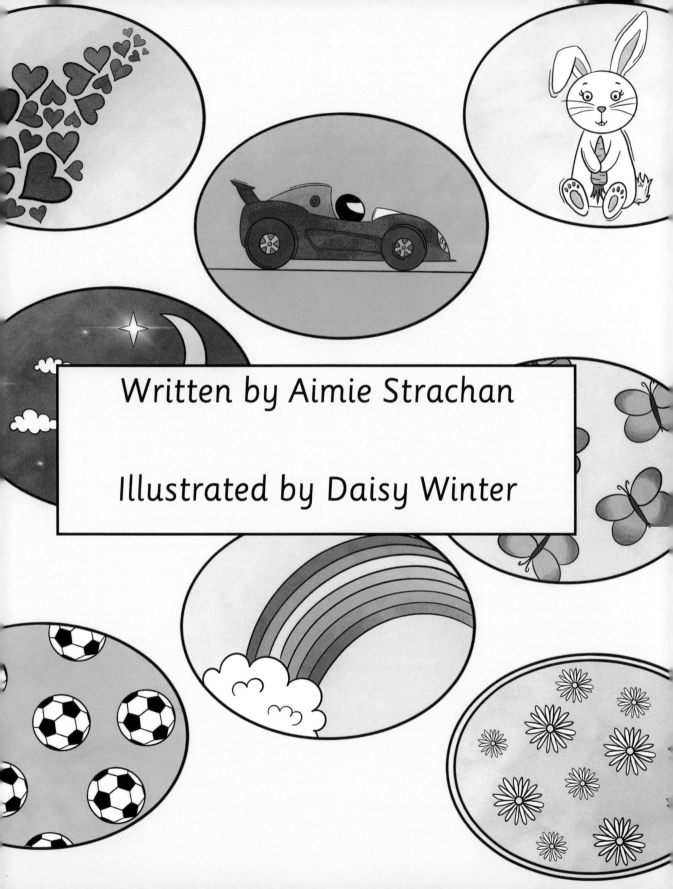

Written by Aimie Strachan

Illustrated by Daisy Winter

My name is Matilda.

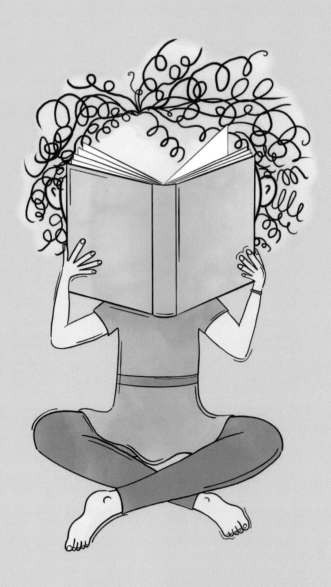

I like reading.

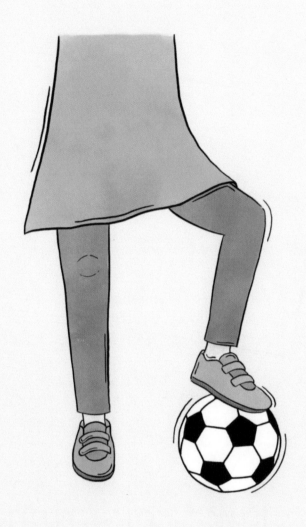

I like playing football.

I like colouring.

I wear glasses to help
me see better.

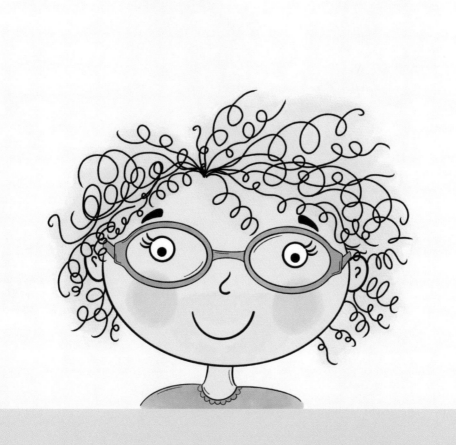

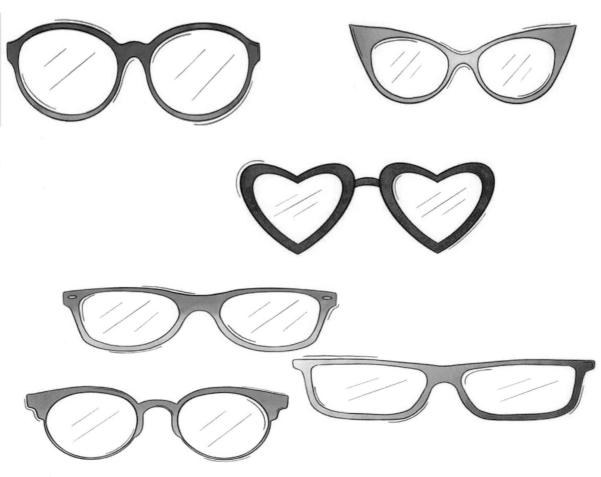

Which glasses do you
like best?

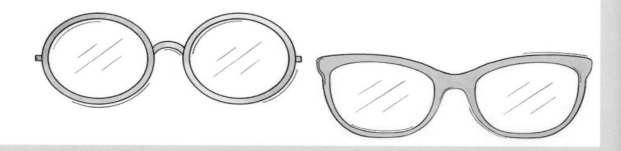

To check my eyes I visit an Orthoptist. I have to wear funny glasses. Things go a bit blurry.

(An Orthoptist specialises in diagnosing and treating visual problems involving eye movement and alignment.)

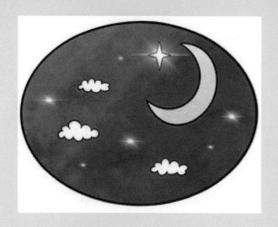 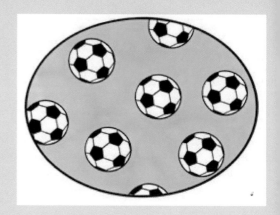

One of my eyes needs a bit of extra help to work better.

I get to choose an eye patch to make my eye stronger.

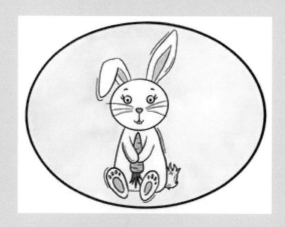

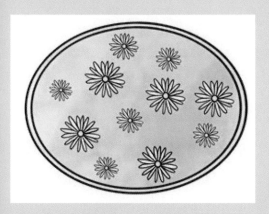
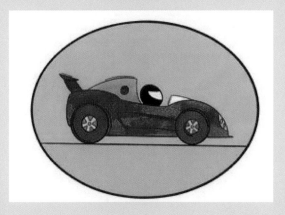

Which eye patch
would you choose?

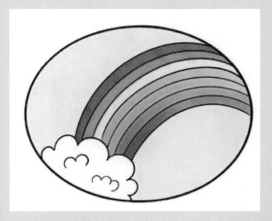
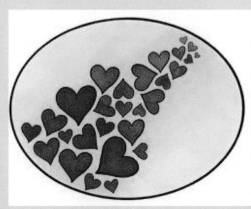
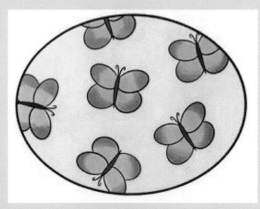

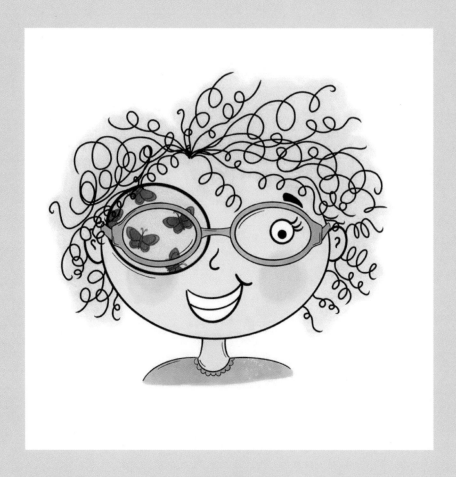

I am very excited for Mummy to put the eye patch on.

At first it is a bit strange and I can't see Mummy.

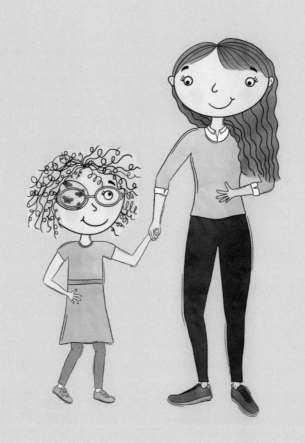

Then she stands in front of me and my eye can see more clearly.

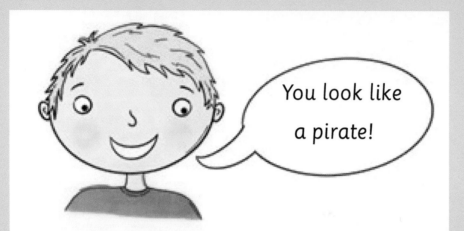

Wearing an eye patch makes me feel special!

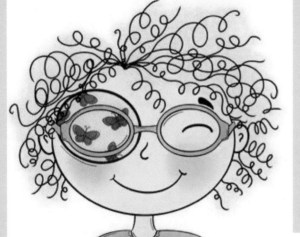

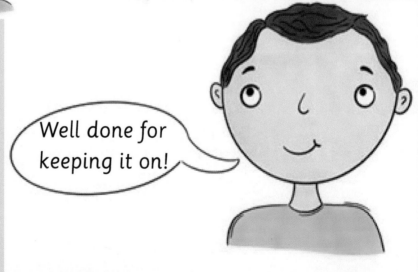

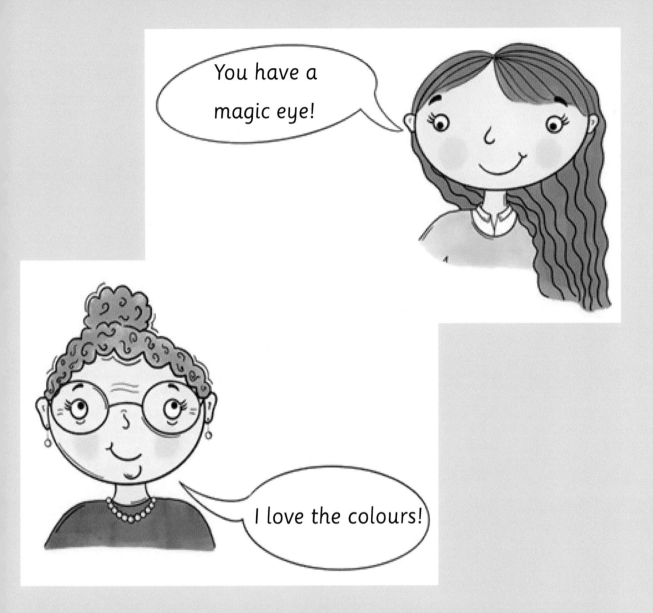

The Orthoptist says if I wear my eye patch every day, my eye will work better.

Mummy gets me a reward
chart and reminds me
to wear my patch.

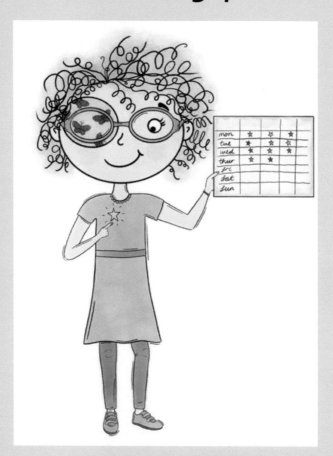

I like getting star stickers.

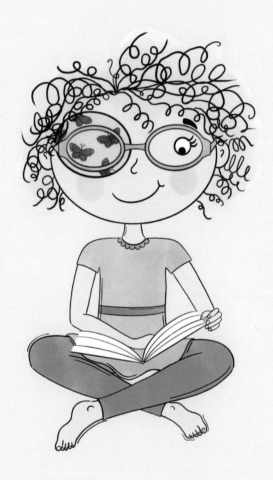

I still like reading.

I still like football.

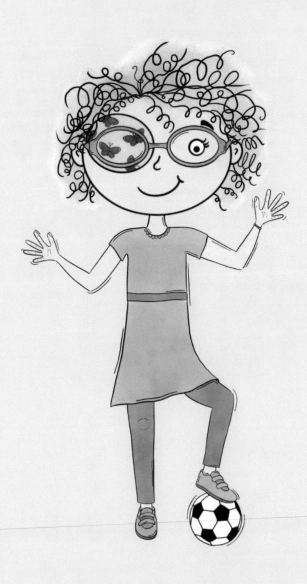

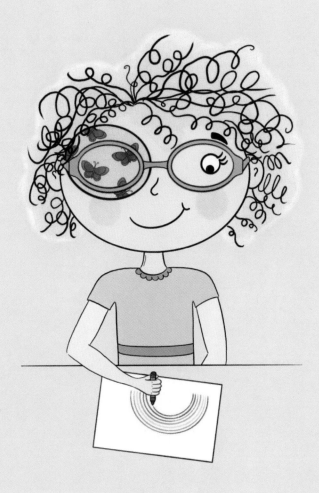

I still like colouring.

And I still like cake!

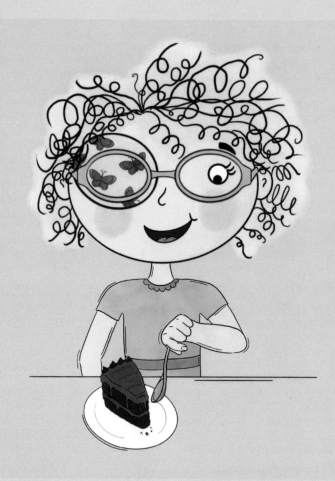

I am still me.

- 1 in 50 children develop a lazy eye (NHS.uk)
- The younger the child is when a lazy eye is diagnosed, the more successful treatment is likely to be. (NHS.uk)

- Patches are most effective before a child reaches 6 years of age (NHS.uk)

- Using a patch involves wearing a patch over the 'good' eye so the lazy eye is forced to work. (NHS.uk)

- Using a patch…can often be an unpleasant experience. This is why the most important thing…to do is explain the reasons for using a patch and the importance of sticking with the treatment to your child so that they're motivated to do it. (NHS.uk)

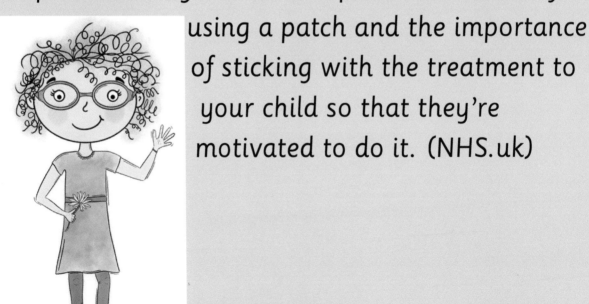

Guide to Patching

When a child patches it is to improve the vision in one eye. The 'good' eye is patched to force the other eye to develop. It must be scary for children when beginning patching so be mindful of this.

1. To begin, patch for a short time using a timer and sitting or playing together. 'Busy hands' activities are a good way to stop patch removal.
2. Keep it positive, always have a smile and praise any patch wearing.
3. Continue through the day, patching for a few minutes at a time.
4. Use a reward chart and let your child choose the stickers.
5. Decide on small rewards and then perhaps something bigger at the end of a period of patching.
6. Let your child choose the patch. Having some ownership will encourage patching.
7. LOTS of verbal praise.
8. Consistency is key. Patch at the same time every day so a routine is established.

Your child will get used to patching. The longer you stick with it, the more the 'weak' eye develops and vision improves.

You're doing it for the right reasons, stick with it!

Printed in Great Britain
by Amazon

20272946R00016